IGNITE YOUR PASSION WITH A
**CASH THERAPY PRACTICE**

ON
FIRE

PAUL POTTER, PT

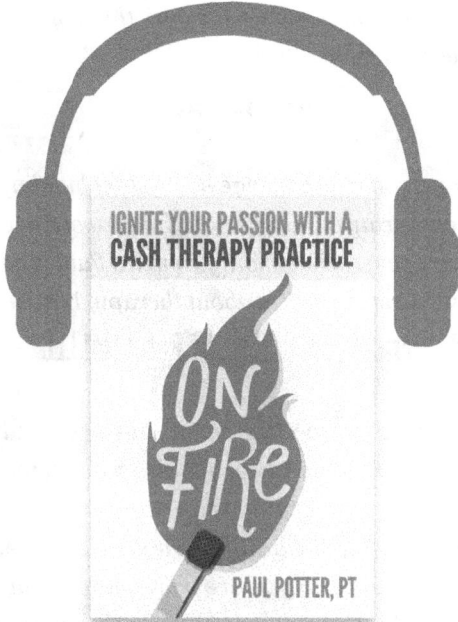

## DOWNLOAD THE AUDIOBOOK FREE!

### READ THIS FIRST

Just to say thank you for purchasing my book, I would like to give
you the audiobook version 100% FREE!

### TO DOWNLOAD

Go to PaulPotterPT.com/freeaudiobook

*"Paul Potter has been my mentor for my business as well as my personal life, guiding me to find the right balance between family and work. Paul has been a successful business owner for over thirty years and has never lost his genuine desire to help others."*

## Jake DeNell PT

*"Paul was the first person to encourage me to start building my own dream practice, which meant transitioning from clinical work to empowering OTs and patients through generating quality content. Paul is a man of character and an encourager. When he writes about therapy, I listen."*

## Sarah Lyon, OTR/L, OT Potential LLC

*"Paul Potter has a broad perspective on life, business, and physical therapy from many years of practice, but also from living a close, disciplined life in Christ. His writing is an expression of his passion for teaching others and sharing the insight he has received. As my friend and mentor, I can assure you that if you are passionate about pursuing a goal with Paul's help, he will honestly and sincerely do whatever he can to assist you in attaining your goal."*

## Zack Zade PT, DPT, CSCS

*"I have known Paul Potter as a man constantly searching for knowledge and understanding and willing to share this newfound information with all who are around him. I also know Paul is a successful and innovative practice owner. He publishes an interesting and informative blog, stays up to date with all the newest social technologies, and continues to improve himself as a therapist and a professional. Paul has asked me to have open blog discussions on a couple of topics over the past few years and always comes to our meetings informed, interested in the materials, and ready to create a deep and meaningful discussion. I look forward to any material he presents within the professional practice arena."*

## Steven W. Forbush, PT, PhD, OCS, CSMT

*"I have known Paul Potter as a friend colleague and brother in Christ for nearly thirty-eight years. He is the kind of person one has to admire. He is passionate about his family, his faith and his profession. Over the years I have observed his commitment to quality and purpose. I am sure that you will be inspired by his vision for turning passion into a cash-based physical therapy practice."*

## Kevin Rippey, PT, MPA

*"Paul exudes energy and encouragement in his interactions, and I have been empowered after every encounter with him. As a leader, he has walked with me through the journey of starting my own practice. As a facilitator, he has helped me draw out my story—something that does not come naturally. As a problem-solver, he has listened and understood, being able to cooperatively define the next step in my journey. He does this with grace and humility, making him a very safe confidant. I am proud to call him a friend."*

## Tom Kruse PT

*"As the CEO of International Spine and Pain Institute, I encounter thousands of healthcare providers annually in the U.S. and internationally at conferences and weekend intensive workshops. This is where I met Paul Potter, a highly driven physical therapist interested in making the world a better place one client at a time. Paul is one of a very small select group of healthcare providers who has dedicated themselves to a higher level of practice, completing our advanced spinal manual therapy certification. Paul is a scholar at heart, always eager to listen, learn and be part of the solution. Paul has continued his growth beyond our organization with care for his clients and growing the profession. Paul is an asset to the physical therapy community and will continue to reach higher and higher."*

## Adriaan Louw, PhD
## CEO International Spine and Pain Institute

# On Fire: Ignite Your Passion with a Cash Therapy Practice
## By Paul Potter, PT

Copyright 2015 by Paul Potter
All Rights Reserved
Published in the United States by Resilient Group Publishing
ISBN-978-0-9963844-1-4

heypaul@paulpotterpt.com
paulpotterpt.com

## The Author

Paul Potter, PT. After 35 years of managing a solo therapy practice, I feel called to share what I've learned with the next generation of therapists. I want to help therapists escape factory-like therapy to create a dream practice. My dream is that this book will help you in your journey towards professional and personal freedom while doing the work you love.

## Dedication

To therapists, who follow their dreams, take risks and have a burning desire to change the world.

# CONTENTS

# PREFACE

Do you feel called to be a therapist? I know I do. As therapists we have tremendous opportunity to use our abilities, education and expertise to enhance clients' lives. What a privilege! If you are in the therapy business to serve people, then this book is for you.

The healthcare landscape has changed dramatically. It can feel like a major earthquake has disrupted everything from how therapists get referrals to how they get paid. Providing transformative therapy has become more difficult as regulations increase and reimbursements decline. These ongoing shifts have left many therapists feeling over worked, overwhelmed and undervalued.

That is the bad news.

The good news is that there is a way to find your footing. Innovative therapists are using alternative ways to deliver the high-value care their clients so desperately need. Cash-based therapy practices have emerged as a viable alternative to accepting business as usual.

In this book, I want to go beyond the typical "copy my model of success" approach. Books written from this perspective, while providing some valuable information and practical advice, fall short. Let me explain why.

To understand what choices you should make about your therapy practice, we need to start with a bird's eye view. A look at the bigger picture will provide perspective on your place in the new healthcare economy. The cash-based therapy model is in its infancy and it will change considerably as it grows and adapts. You must build a business not just for today, but one that is malleable enough to be effective in the future.

The "do what I did" approach has a second short-coming. Most cash-based practices are designed and built upon the needs of an ideal client base and a therapist's unique value proposition. Therefore, no one formula can be applied to every practice and guarantee success. Although every business goes through similar stages of development, each will take a distinct path to reach its destination.

With these things in mind, I've set out to provide a book for those who want to understand the changing healthcare climate and what it means for therapists. *On Fire* explores why old approaches and practices will no longer work. I have provided examples of therapists who have taken the leap to a full cash-based practice to learn from, but I've also included discussions about developing your unique calling and listening to your prospective clients. This will help you discern the route that you—and only you—might take to building a new kind of practice.

To plan your journey I've created a four-part roadmap to walk you through the stages of a small business startup. These aren't the stages that your practice will automatically go through. They are the stages that your business *should* go through for the best opportunity for success.

I've worked with and learned from many successful therapists during my 35-year career as a private practice owner. In this book I've combined the wisdom of the past with new entrepreneurial strategies to prepare you for the challenges of building a profitable business.

The difference between a successful practice and a failed one is clarity on your destination, having a sense of direction and taking the next step. In this book I lay out the four stages to building a successful practice including road signs to look for and detours to avoid.

At the end of the book there is a link to resources and tools to help you get started on your journey.

In my conversations with therapists I've found four fears that sometimes prevent them from pursuing a dream practice:

### 1. Marketing
They just aren't confident in their ability to connect with and book more clients. The dreaded four-letter word S-E-L-L causes many therapists to settle for the status quo.

### 2. Business
Many therapists confess they don't know how to run a business to make a profit.

### 3. Mastery.
Other therapists lack confidence in their clinical expertise and shrink from operating on their own.

### 4. Technology.
Therapists say they feel uncertain about and overwhelmed by the technology needed to run a modern business.

If any of these fears sound familiar, perhaps *On Fire* will be a spark of inspiration and guidance.

Therapists who have overcome their trepidation have experienced a sense of liberation. They have moved from being victims of the shifting landscape to successful entrepreneurs who experience:

### 1. Personal Freedom
### 2. Professional Freedom
### 3. Financial Freedom

You will get value from just reading this book. But, just like our therapy clients, the true value occurs when you take an active role. You must put your new knowledge into action. Write out your answers to the questions. Record your personal action steps with deadlines and do them.

It will take courage to pursue your calling, take action and move toward the kind of freedom innovative therapists are beginning to experience. I didn't set out to write a book about courage, but the deeper I've looked into what it takes to build a cash-based practice, the more clearly I've seen that it takes courage to choose to act differently. Without courage, all the instruction on business and growth is just so many notes on white boards or in binders. I say this without judgment because fear is a part of being human. Courage is not the absence of fear but the will to act in the midst of fear.

## What compels us beyond fear is simply going back to that very first question: Do you feel called to be a therapist?

People in your community need your unique service now. These are the people you are called to serve. Don't miss this opportunity. Don't settle for going about business as usual while clinging to the vague hope the things will get better on their own. If you do, you'll miss your calling and many wonderful people will miss the comfort and healing you can provide.

# INTRODUCTION: ON FIRE

For those of you who want to kiss corporate therapy goodbye and create your dream practice, I have some good news. A growing number of therapists have ignited their passion for quality care and professional freedom. I urge you to join these smart, motivated therapists who are creating new ways to deliver quality, client-focused care.

In the old healthcare economy most therapists were part of a supply chain in large, vertically integrated organizations. Because of the massive capital requirements and economies of scale required to be competitive, many organizations merged into even larger corporate silos.

Fee-for-service models permitted extensive corporate expansion and profitability. All players, including therapists, were content with this arrangement because there seemed to be plenty of money to go around. For those healthcare providers seeking professional autonomy, private practice was always an option. For the most part, however, private practices operated by the same rules as everyone else. Times have changed. Contentment with the status quo is threatening the core identity and clinical practice of rehabilitation professionals.

In the new healthcare economy, every therapist needs to be an entrepreneur. Embracing an entrepreneurial mindset provides the best chance of achieving professional freedom while doing the work you love. The Internet has made this option both viable and attractive.

You may have noticed that the world is a vastly different place since the Internet went mainstream. Easy access to health information and global connectivity has brought about a revolution in the way healthcare is delivered and consumed.

The Internet has created opportunity for thousands of small, independent businesses to operate outside the domination of the gigantic healthcare corporations. The playing field has shifted in favor of small, agile physical therapy practices that are in direct contact with the direct users of healthcare. The Internet allows consumers to be more educated and empowered when they seek medical services. Innovative therapists have seen the writing on the wall and chosen to take this moment to take control of their careers.

A growing number of therapists are capitalizing on the new mantra that "small is better." They have abandoned hierarchical corporate therapy to create indie therapy practices. Technology has made it possible for therapists to have direct access to patients, outsource office support, and automate repetitive tasks. Indie clinics with drastically reduced overhead and personalized care are able to effectively compete with the big boys. Entrepreneurs are siphoning business away from obsolete incumbents as they move into new markets with cost-sensitive solutions.

It is my hope that this book will spark inspiration, ingenuity and inventiveness in every therapist who reads it.

## If you yearn to rekindle the fire for your therapy career and learn about the new business of therapy, read on.

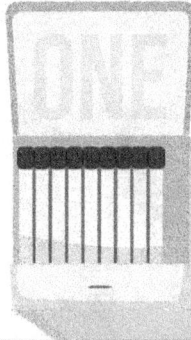

# PART ONE

## CALLING

*You don't "just know" what your calling is. You must listen for clues along the way, discovering what your life can tell you. Awareness comes with practice.*

*–Jeff Goines*

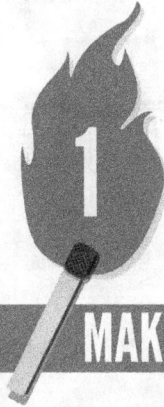

# CHAPTER ONE / MAKE A DIFFERENCE

I wrote this book based upon three premises:

1. You are on earth to make a difference in the lives of the people you are called to serve. Serving others through professional therapy is a noble calling.

2. Your expertise, experience and unique talent are the best way to transform lives and are of greater value than you realize.

3. You can build a dream practice that provides you with both the professional and personal freedom to live a deeply meaningful life.

I do not have a double blind study in a peer-reviewed journal to prove any of my premises, so if you remain skeptical, I don't blame you. I do know that you are bombarded daily with negative messages that challenge your professional self-esteem:

- Unnecessary denials from insurance companies
- Patient no-shows
- Physicians demanding patients see their in-house therapists
- Endless documentation requiring proof of client improvement.

Cost containment has become the goal in the chaotic, rapidly changing medical environment. Third-party payers often see therapy as more of a liability than an asset. We must not allow insurance networks, government regulations or managed care to undermine our value or dismiss the significant contribution we make to our patients' welfare. This relentless scrutiny can distort our self-perception and confidence.

In reality, the therapy community is a group of caring professionals who serve people with their knowledge and hands-on care. We are empathetic experts who desire respect and to be paid fairly for the value we deliver. We are ordinary individuals doing extraordinary things every day. We transform our patients' lives. We are good at what we do. We make a positive difference in the world.

If this is true, why do so many therapists describe feeling undervalued, overworked and unfulfilled? Just attend a professional conference and you sense a quiet desperation from colleagues as they talk about their jobs. Many therapists have lost their passion and vision for their careers. When I talk with therapists about patient care, however, I get the sense that most of them still love the art of therapy and working with clients. Most still have a hunger to learn, to improve their skills and to excel at what they do. Some have dreams of owning their own clinics where they will have freedom to practice the way they want and with whom they want. Before I suggest how you might successfully accomplish these goals, I want to talk about a key principle that can unlock your potential to soar to new heights—A Growth Mindset.

## Growth Mindset

Deep in your gut you know that, given a fair chance, you can make a significant difference in the lives of your patients. You're confident that your knowhow and skills have been instrumental in your clients' before-and-after transformations. You may not see yourself as an expert or an extraordinary therapist, but merely as someone doing what needs to be done, sometimes at a personal sacrifice. In other words, just doing your job.

Unfortunately, if these beliefs are held too tightly they will encumber you in the new healthcare economy. From her twenty years of research, Carol S. Dweck, Ph.D. discovered that the view people adopt for themselves profoundly affects the way they lead their lives. In her book *Mindset*, she categorizes self-belief into two distinct mindsets, fixed and growth.

With a fixed mindset you believe that your qualities are carved in stone. Believing you only have a certain amount of intelligence, a certain degree of professional effectiveness and therefore a certain value, you'll find yourself having to validate your worth again and again. I've seen many therapists consumed with trying to prove themselves to patients, peers and physicians.

Contrast that desperation for approval with a growth mindset. A growth mindset is based upon the belief that your basic qualities are things you can cultivate through your efforts. Why waste time and effort proving yourself to an often fickle and uncaring audience when you could be focusing on professional improvement? Why look to traditional referral sources to prop up your self-esteem instead of building your own relationship with potential clients? A growth mindset permits you to stretch yourself, especially during the challenges of building up a practice.

You may be asking yourself why others don't seem to recognize and appreciate your expertise. Could your insecurities be the main reason? Are you putting your dreams on hold not because of external circumstances but because of your own mindset? Are you afraid of offending the doctor who sends you patients? Are you competing with and comparing yourself to other therapists? Are you holding yourself back until you get more training or advanced certifications to prove to yourself and others that you are good enough? This book will challenge you to move beyond these mental obstacles. We will focus on those things that are under your influence and learn ways to let go of the factors outside of your control. A cash therapy practice startup really begins with the startup of you.

## Abundance Mindset

Once you've committed yourself to a growth mindset, you will then be able to transfer that proactive thinking to the marketplace. Ultimately, it is the marketplace that determines the value of your services. The worth of your services is what people are willing to pay for with their time, money and effort. This is where the rubber meets the road.

Author Stephen Covey (*The Seven Habits of Highly Effective People*) conceived the idea of an abundance mindset. In this concept a person believes that there are sufficient resources and successes to go around. Covey contrasts this perspective with a scarcity mindset, which infers that if someone else wins, you lose. Therapists with an abundance mentality reject the notion of the zero-sum game. They believe there is an abundance of people in the world who need to be served. They are able to celebrate the success of others rather than feel threatened by it.

If you possess an abundance mindset, you will see opportunities for growth where others see threats. You will be willing to form new relationships with nontraditional partners. You will be generous with your knowledge and resources because you believe that the pie is big enough for everyone. You will not be distracted by who gets the biggest piece of pie because you are focused on growth and serving your customers.

As therapists, we have the training and the skills to provide a valuable service for which people are willing to pay. We have allowed third-party middlemen to distort our value to the consumer. It's time to get back in touch with people who desperately need our services. It is to your benefit to sell— yes, I said sell—your services directly to the consumer. Listening directly to the healthcare consumer is the key to offering affordable services to meet their true healthcare needs. A growth mindset allows cash therapy providers to go directly to their ideal clients and exchange value for value. It's a win-win attitude and one you can learn.

Many therapists have been brainwashed into a dependence on physicians for permission to work with clients. Your mindset is the starting point for you to see yourself as an equal member of the healthcare team. If you don't believe in your value then others won't either.

Each of us brings different aptitudes, experiences and temperaments to our careers. Scientists are discovering we have much more potential for brain development and lifelong learning than previously imagined. Your intelligence and professional skill are not fixed quantities. Lifelong learning and practice improves your clinical competency. Expertise empowers you to escape the medical hierarchy to stand on your professional effectiveness.

To grow you are going to have to take steps that are out of your comfort zone. I mean really out of your comfort zone, to the point where it hurts and it's scary. It's easy to stick with the familiar, but comfort rarely leads to excellence.

The purpose of *On Fire* is to help you get out of your comfort zone, push through the challenges and pursue your calling. We are going to look at why the old way of doing therapy doesn't work anymore. I'll share my struggle to discover and live out my calling. We'll then dive into the changing healthcare economy, and discover how to thrive in it. The book concludes with mistakes to avoid, steps necessary to build a successful cash therapy practice and resources to help with the process.

**You've made it through the first chapter so if you want a fresh take on thriving in the new healthcare economy read on.**

# PRIMARY CARE MINDSET

## Aaron LeBauer PT, DPT, LMBT

What would be your mindset if the largest multispecialty practice in your region had your grandfather's name and picture on the building?

This is the scenario that faced Aaron LeBauer as he set up his cash-based therapy practice in Greensboro, North Carolina. Aaron's father and several of his uncles are physicians. Two months after graduating as a Doctor of Physical Therapy, Aaron faced an important decision: How was he was going to view himself as he promoted his practice? He had an advantage over his classmates because he had run a successful massage therapy practice prior to PT school. He knew the pitfalls of the physician-gatekeeper model and the benefits of direct access to his massage therapy clients. He chose from the outset to view himself as a primary care provider.

Aaron believes that mindset is everything. He strongly encourages therapists to cultivate a primary care mindset and to market directly to patients. Since 2008, Aaron and his wife have successfully operated a 100% cash-based practice by providing a high-value service and forming a direct payment relationship with clients.

**Aaron is a free-spirited pioneer who introduces himself to his patients by saying, "I am Doctor LeBauer and I am your physical therapist." He believes and projects that he is a primary care physical therapist and a musculoskeletal expert. Gradually, his word of mouth referrals have far surpassed the traditional referral sources.**

Dr. LeBauer helps other therapists start cash-based therapy practices through his writing, videoconferences and consultations at LeBauerConsulting.com.

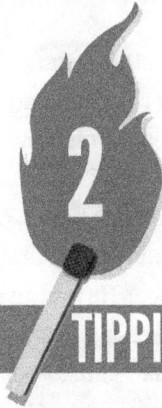

# CHAPTER TWO / TIPPING POINT

In 2006, author Malcolm Gladwell created a tipping point of his own when he wrote his book, *The Tipping Point*. The book's premise is that small changes can eventually make a significant difference. When small numbers of people act differently, the cumulative effect increases until a critical point or "tipping point" is reached. The term tipping point is frequently used to describe social behavior in business, especially the word-of-mouth viral spread of an idea or consumer behavior.

Leaders in healthcare, government and business believe that the U.S. healthcare system is at a tipping point. Reformers hope that recent changes have the healthcare system heading in a positive direction. They are hedging their bets that society has learned from the past as well as from the experience of other countries. Naysayers point to the failure of the Affordable Care Act's website and the liquidation of CoOportunity Health as proof that we are sliding backwards to higher costs and poorer quality healthcare. Whether positive or negative, there is no question that healthcare delivery and reimbursement are undergoing fundamental changes.

For several decades, healthcare providers have endured various solutions to the healthcare crisis only to experience more regulations and paperwork for less reimbursement and time with patients. Many therapists have grown skeptical towards any news of impending change.

A majority of therapists sense that system corrections are inevitable. A few are planning now to be ahead of the curve. They would prefer not to deal with monumental changes in the reimbursement system all at once. Farsighted leaders are preparing for bundled payments, pay-for-performance and capitation fees, to name a few. The issue for therapists is how and when to be proactive.

## Left Behind

You don't want to be left behind in the aftermath of change. You want to be riding the wave rather than struggling to keep your head above water. But be honest with yourself. How do you usually respond to change?

*Crossing the Chasm,* by Geoffrey A. Moore describes an adoption life cycle. In this classic work about embracing new technology, Moore describes the responses to innovation divided across five segments of the classic bell curve. These categories are identified as innovators, early adopters, early majority, late majority and laggards. Where do you fit?

What makes the early adopters so different from the majority is the reason why they buy into a new idea or concept. They are buying into change itself and into the opportunity to get a jump on the competition. They expect a significant shift in their industry. They believe the old ideas, strategies and rules are quickly on the way out and will be replaced by the new.

The early majority is looking for improvements in existing system. They do not want to mess around with products and systems that haven't been perfected, or to master new innovations that can't be integrated into the existing way of doing things.

On the far right of the bell curve are the laggards who resist change at all costs. They are more comfortable with life as it is or wish they could go back to their idea of the good old days.

The point I want to make with the adoption life cycle is that it is important to honestly assess your natural reaction to change. Equally important is understanding how quickly the market where you practice adapts to change. You may not want to unleash an innovative new practice in a slow-adapting marketplace.

Your perception of change will determine your ability to see new realities. Where you fall on Moore's curve effects your motivation to acquire new knowledge and skills. The downside to lagging behind the curve is you're always trying to catch up while working against the momentum of change.

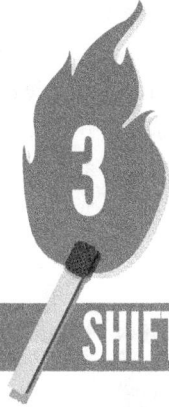

# CHAPTER THREE    SHIFT HAPPENS

When individuals are subject to too much change in too little time, they experience what Alvin Toffler called future shock. All the change brought about by healthcare reform and increased regulations can lead to the shattering stress and disorientation described by Toffler. You can take your pick from the alphabet soup of new regulations: PQRS, FLR, or G-codes. There has been wave after wave of change in reimbursements, organizational mergers and increased efforts to reduce fraud and waste.

The effects of this fundamental reshaping of healthcare are no longer only being felt at an administrative level.  Healthcare reform has worked its way down to main street rehabilitation services. Future shock is here.

Instinctively, I want to hunker down in a safe, quiet harbor somewhere and wait for the storm to pass. I just want to be left alone to practice therapy in a manner that helps patients get better. Believe me, I know the cost of healthcare in this country. I'm self-employed and I've watched my health insurance skyrocket for the last three decades. I've watched first hand as my patients' deductibles and copays have steadily increased while their benefits have decreased.

## No Safe Harbors

The reality is, whether you work in a large hospital or in a small clinic, there is no quiet harbor or Gilligan's Island far away from the disruptions in modern medicine. Everyone is effected when change happens within an industry as large as healthcare. System theory says that any change in one component part of a system affects people in all other parts of the system.

So it is not a matter of whether or not therapy as we know it will change, but more about how we are going to adapt to change. This quote from Sydney J. Harris describes the internal paradox many of us may be feeling:

**"Our dilemma is that we hate change and love it at the same time; what we really want is for things to remain the same but to get better."**

Every change involves some type of loss, as well as a new beginning. When we are required to transform our work it often means giving up old habits and comfortable routines.

One of the most important steps in making the transition from old to new is to understand the emotional process we go through when dealing with change. Change is situational and often outside of our control. Transition, on the other hand, is a process that temporarily or permanently changes your routine or life. Transition is under your control. Your mindset during a transition is often based upon your feelings of self-esteem and your abilities to deal with change.

This is where I see therapists get stuck. Change can be perceived as either positive or negative. Change may be the result of a choice that you have made or it may be from unwanted mandates over which you have no control. Whatever the source of the change, how you process your emotions is key in moving forward. I find myself slipping back into wishing for the past when life in the clinic was less complicated. If I'm not careful I find myself holding on to the way things used to be and not taking steps toward the future.

Every transition will require letting go of the old way of doing things, establishing new routines for getting your work done and feeling good about it. You have to release the familiar to grab hold of the new. If you have a death grip on the way you've always done things, you'll never be able to learn the new ways required by the ever-changing system. Easier said than done.

## Good Grief

An important step in letting go of your previous identity as a therapist is to allow yourself to grieve what has been lost. Good grief is embracing the emotions that naturally occur when there has been a significant change or loss. You'll experience a variety of normal human emotions as you process change. An understanding of the emotional steps involved in processing grief can be very helpful. Feelings like shock, denial, anger, depression or guilt can be experienced in varying degrees. We may have experienced co-workers who became negative, cynical or depressed as a reaction to the recent changes in healthcare. This may be part of the normal process of grieving.

To grow as a person or an organization we must go through transitional experiences to get to the other side of change. Within these experiences are victories and setbacks of life. Change and transition are an integral and necessary part of life. Although comprehension of the emotional stages won't alleviate experiencing the emotions themselves, it will go a long way in helping you overcome the fear and disorientation that often occurs.

You might find it beneficial to take a moment to remember previous transitions that you've walked through. Recall how you felt during those periods of remarkable change and transition. How did you deal with the emotions of denial, anxiety or anger? What did you say to yourself during those times of transition? Did you use self-talk phrases such as "I can do this" or "This is stupid, it will never work"?

If you got angry, where or towards whom did you direct your anger? Did you direct it at people who were not involved in your situation? Did you vent your frustrations to others who had no power to influence the situation? If you got depressed or buried your emotions, what did you do to cope? Was it healthy or was it an escape that diverted you from making progress?

Most healthcare providers have recently experienced an immense amount of change in a short period of time. Many are struggling to catch their breath just when the next round of changes begins. Letting go of the old ways, walking through the in-between phase, then growing comfortable with your new situation is all a part of the process. Relying on the skills you learned while processing change in the past will guide you as you transition or pivot into your new identity and sense of purpose.

## Pivot

One way to assert control in the midst of the chaos of change is to choose when to pivot. Be a student of your industry so you can choose when to make your own change.

Professions, like businesses, follow a predictable life cycle. Some might call it morbid for therapists to analyze the overall health of their profession. Where does the therapy profession, particularly private practice, fall in its professional lifecycle? Is it on the rise, has it matured, or is it in a decline? Is the marketplace crowded and the market demand for your services falling off? If traditional therapy is dying a slow death, then it is time for life saving resuscitation. In the business startup world this is often called pivoting. Keeping one foot on the ground while you shift weight and change your direction. Maybe the writing is on the wall in your present job and you need a career pivot.

I've slightly modified Josh Linkner's article from *Forbes* magazine, "When to Pivot: 7 Signs Your Company is Dying," to help you determine if you should pivot from your present job.

1. The same results require double the effort. You as a therapist find yourself mired in non-productive bureaucracy and not maximizing your expertise. Effectiveness and efficiency are the hallmarks of a service that's on the rise.
2. The team has lost its swagger. When therapists enjoy and are passionate about their work the energy is obvious. Clients and other team members feed off this energy and it generates results.
3. You deliver more excuses than results. As referrals and numbers drop you blame outside factors. You hear more complaining than creativity. Blaming isn't going to change anything. If you want to be

the captain of your own career then you must take responsibility to steer it.

4. You believe the market and tech trends don't apply to your business. Therapists have been guilty of this mindset for years. Third-party payer reimbursement in healthcare is slowly changing to a pay-for-performance system. No matter how good you are, the market will eventually determine the value of your services. You shouldn't base your practice in a vacuum independent of marketplace factors.

Pivoting in any organization is difficult, but especially in today's environment of warp-speed reform and increasing competition. It is imperative that therapists keep nimble on their feet, able to change directions in their career. Pivoting involves keeping your center of balance around your core. Your decision on when to take action should be based upon your core values and assets. Thoughtful and careful planning is key to a successful implementation.

Sometimes, however, life can be cruel. It can throw you a curve ball. The world is under no obligation to make your dreams come true. Hard times will come. It's during these moments that we are tempted to give up, but they provide us the opportunity to dig deep and be more intentional than ever.

In the next chapter I'll share how I faced a major health crisis in my life and, out of desperation, pivoted my career in a whole new direction.

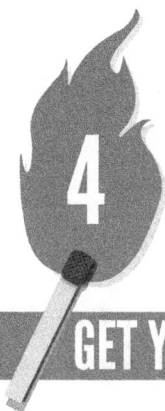

# CHAPTER FOUR — GET YOUR HOUSE IN ORDER

"Paul, my advice to you is that you better get your house in order." These were the words that Dave, a physician friend, said to me.

I remember the sickness I felt in the pit of my stomach as my wife and I drove home from Dave's house. I vividly remember the overwhelming fear. That night I realized what a panic attack was. I just couldn't relax. I absolutely couldn't go to sleep.

It was on that night that I came to grips with the diagnosis that the surgeon had given me two weeks earlier. It was that night that I was shocked out of my denial that I had cancer. It was then that I had to deal with my own mortality and purpose in life.

Let me give you the backstory. My wife and I had moved back to Lincoln, Nebraska, so I could earn my master's degree and we could be near friends and family. I began an outpatient therapy practice from scratch during the last year of graduate school. I worked in the business one or two days per week while also holding down a part-time job at the hospital. I started out with one small room, a desk, my head and my hands.

Over a period of 10 years the practice and our family grew. I was able to move into a new space for my practice and hire a couple of employees. My wife, Anne, was able to leave her job as a therapist to care for our children.

Anne delivered our fourth daughter. In anticipation of outgrowing our rental, we built a new house. The practice had produced well over a five-year period of time and we had saved enough to build our dream home. With great excitement and joy we move into our new home with three little girls and a baby. We were connected with other families in our church with young children and were homeschooling our older daughters. Life was good.

Since I owned my business I had the freedom to pursue my passions. I believed in the value of wellness, so early on I integrated a fitness center into my practice. I made time to spend with my children and time to invest in other men who needed a mentor, an encourager or just a friend. It was a busy, challenging, but fulfilling time. I was living my dream as a husband, father and solo practitioner. Little did I know that my dream was about to turn into my worst nightmare.

## Life is Not a Dream

Right after we had moved into our new home I felt a lump in my armpit. I thought nothing of it for months, assuming it would go away. I thought it was probably just a swollen lymph node from some type of infection. I prided myself on my health. I ran marathons, played college basketball and heck, I had my master's degree in wellness. I regularly practiced many spiritual disciplines. I soon learned, though, that even wellness experts are human and vulnerable.

The lump didn't go away. It was surgically removed and sent off to pathology. I remember the day I returned to the surgeon's office to get the lab report. The strange, fearful look on the receptionist's face should have been a tip off. Ironically, while I waited I was reading Steven Covey's time management book, *First Things First*. I kid you not.

The surgeon came in and quickly delivered the bad news. "Paul, the pathology report came back and you've been diagnosed with stage three malignant melanoma." I was shocked. I was caught completely off guard. He didn't know what to do next and I didn't know what to do with myself. I could hardly think.

I had patients to see in my clinic after my appointment. I had no one else. I was the practice. I drove back to my clinic and finished out the day. I told my staff. My wife and I cried together sitting on the floor of our bedroom closet away from our four little daughters. I was in a fog. A cancer fog would be with me on a daily basis for the next five years.

Shortly after the diagnosis, my doctor told me that my odds of survival where at best one in a thousand. I was told that I might have as little as a year to live and to get my house in order. I had to face the question that is often asked in a theoretical sense: "If you were told you had one year to live, what would you do?"

Here I was as a 40-year-old with a wife, four small children and my own business. It wasn't a theoretical mission statement exercise. It was my reality.

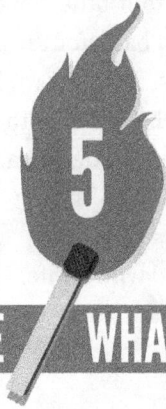

# CHAPTER FIVE / WHAT'S YOUR WHY?

This is my story. I've learned to share it with greater detail over the years. In the beginning I was afraid to even talk about having a terminal diagnosis. I was more comfortable denying it was real and hoping it was a bad dream.

I have heard people talk of being diagnosed with cancer as a gift. I slowly began to understand what they meant. It changed how I looked at life. The malignancy made me appreciate the precious relationships I had with my family. It made me face my own mortality head on and live for what counted the most in this life and the life after. Since my life might end any day, I wanted to live for what was transcendent. I wanted to live without any regrets.

No regrets of not dreaming big, of not taking risks or of missing out on simple memories with my loved ones. I was going out fighting and not holding anything back.

I closed down my practice, simplified my life and focused on strengthening my immune system to fight off the cancer. My wife was unbelievably supportive despite being under considerable stress. The thought of being a young widow with four young children was overwhelming. We pulled each other up as we chose to live in the moment and not in fear of the future.

As months went by I was faced with the practical dilemma of what to do to make a living. I wasn't dead yet and I needed to provide for my family. At the same time, I didn't want to do just any job, but to do work that could be meaningful and could make a difference.

## Course Correction

I hope that the lessons I learned when I weathered my storm will be helpful to you as you think about your own life. A pivot point in your life can be powerful because it takes away all of your excuses. It is not settling for a fall back plan. It's a course correction. Too many times when we suffer a setback we get stuck in "what could have been" or "if only". Life is full of surprises and it won't help us in any way if we live in our past regrets.

At some point you probably entertained the thought that you were going to do something significant as a therapist. You went to college, got good grades, beat the odds and were accepted into therapy school. You survived, graduated and then launched your career with your first therapy job.

Then somewhere along the line the real world set in and you gave up on your dream. Everywhere you went, therapists were making excuses for not doing something extraordinary. Some said they were too busy while others shrugged their shoulders with indifference saying they would figure it out when they grew up. Simple comments like these are hardly insignificant. They grow on you and, like a disease, rob you of your strength. At moments like these, if we don't dig deep down to our core values, we run the risk of abandoning our dreams.

## Calling

I want to help you do the hard work of following your calling to serve others. Discovering your calling can be a struggle and somewhat mysterious.

I call the strong pull or desire to launch out into something purposeful a calling. It is personal. It is about the unique impact you are meant to make in the world through your experience and personality. Discovering your calling happens over time as you walk along the way. It isn't a fixed destination. It's a process in which you are engaged, but it is also something that happens to you. Sometimes it seems it is an internal process that you work through. And at other times it seems to be something outside of you.

You will find calling referred to in many ways. Some people will use the word passion. Some people will call it your life's work. Rick Warren of Saddleback Church defined it as the purpose driven life. I am drawn to the term vocation. Vocation is defined as a strong feeling of suitability for a particular career or occupation.

Before the sixteenth century the term vocation had a much richer, deeper meaning than simply what you did to make a living. In a classical meaning, vocation referred primarily to the call by God on an individual to a particular way of life. The concept of vocation is based upon the Christian belief that God has created each person with a unique set of gifts and talents. Each person is to use these gifts to glorify God by performing his work or calling within the kingdom of God on earth.

Today we use the term passion in place of vocation. Now we speak of work as something that you do to pay the bills. Your passion is what you do from your core being or soul. Your passion is something that excites you. It's something that you love to do. Your passion is an activity that you must do, even if it's not practical, even if you don't get paid for it. As a matter of fact, most of the time you have to pay to engage in your passion.

So the question is can your passion and your career come together as your calling? Can it give you the sense that you are working at what you were made to do? I urge you to see your vocation in the classical point of view. Begin to consider your therapy career as your significant life's work. You might stay at the same employment or you might develop a niche practice, but having a vocation mindset can transform your work experience.

> **"Your calling is not always easy. It will take work. Practice can teach you what you are and are not meant to do."**
> **Jeff Goins, The Art of Work**

It is popular in the current self-help business literature to emphasize a laser-beam focus on identifying your passion in a clearly articulated mission statement. More often than not, unfortunately, life just doesn't cooperate. My process of discovering my calling hasn't been so neat and controlled.

Don't get me wrong. I've written several mission statements, purpose statements, value statements or whatever the current terms are these days. I've just found that life gets messy. I often see more clearly in the rear view mirror than I do looking out the windshield. As we take steps together to develop your professional brand based upon your calling I'd like to have you look for clues in a couple of less obvious places: Mentors whom you've learned from and everyday experiences that have helped you develop as a person.

## Mentors

Mentoring is a word that is thrown out there quite a bit these days when talking about the people and programs that help you develop your professional skills. Therapists are often "mentored" through the professional residencies and internships that have been created to fill the gap between entry-level graduation skills and clinical mastery. Most likely, you want something more in terms of mentoring. You want a person or people who will take a personal interest in your growth and development.

The actual practice of mentoring is difficult to execute properly. Why? Partly because the volume of information has exponentially multiplied, but mostly because mentorship is between people; people who have flaws, who have their own agendas, and who don't live up to ideal expectation. Unknowingly, apprentices can bring Star Wars like expectations of a Yoda mentor. The ideal mentor has the force within and is devoted entirely to helping the trainee develop into a Jedi warrior able to fight the evil empire.

To avoid the idealism trap, let's expand our definition of a mentor to include the wide variety of people you have learned from over your entire life. Think of the parents, teachers and coaches who have helped you get to this point in your life. Chances are that your dream mentor doesn't exist, and if you hold out for this type of teacher you might miss out on important life lessons.

My point is that you can learn something new from virtually everyone you meet in your career journey, both good and bad. Sometimes you can learn the most from supervisors and co-workers who rub against your rough edges. One of the most important characteristics that you can have is a teachable spirit. It seems if someone has a genuine teachable attitude, they can learn from almost every circumstance. I could be a talented therapist with great people skills in a modern clinic with the latest equipment, but if I'm not teachable I will not grow.

I'm surprised at the number of therapists I've met who become defensive with the slightest criticism or correction. They are overly sensitive to negative patient feedback and constructive criticism from their peers. This insecurity prevents many therapists from learning from their mistakes, only to make the same mistakes over and over.

I encourage you to be on the lookout for the unexpected mentors. Each person you work with serves a purpose to help you along your way. Some will offer a tip or small piece of advice. Others will have empathy for your struggles and offer you encouragement and support. If you can see these people as mentors that help you along your path of self-discovery. It will take some of the angst out of always searching for the ideal mentor who can provide everything that you need whenever you need it the most.

A master clinician who is willing and able to mentor you is probably not going to fall into your lap. Try to see that every place you work and every person you meet provides you with a chance to gain clarity on your calling. If nothing else, certain jobs help you to determine what you don't want to do. While I was earning my master's degree, I worked in a university health center with athletes and college students. There I realized the time commitment required to work with athletes. The hours spent in the training room, required attendance at practice and competitive events was a cost I wasn't willing to pay. It wasn't until my desire for sports medicine was put to the test that I discovered my real passion was to help both athletes and non-athletes perform at their best through lifetime fitness.

## Intentional Practice

The other source I'd like you to look at when you are in the process of developing your calling is learning from practicing your profession. This is an area where I see many therapists, particularly young therapists, get hung up on. You can become impatient to let your calling develop over time and hesitant to commit to a career direction. Sometimes the anxiety of making a wrong choice or not appearing as competent as those around you can get the better of you. Impatience can lead to belief that it is different or better somewhere else. To some extent, the manner in which therapists are educated is at fault. The dependence on didactic dissemination of information to large groups of students without real world application creates a gap between knowledge and mastery. There can be an over-reliance on knowledge and less on learning from a master clinician.

Growth as a professional takes time. A therapist's clinical knowledge and skill develops with repetition and practice. It takes years of intentional practice to develop proficiency and mastery. I envy the apprenticeship process of other trades such as plumbers and electricians where they learn as an apprentice under a master craftsman. An electrical apprentice, for example, is typically trained for five years, gradually taking on more responsibility and difficult challenges. Then the apprentice advances to a journeyman for additional years of guided training before graduating to the master level. Now that's the way to master a skill. Deliberate practice under someone who is wiser and more skilled is necessary for high-level mastery. When the sole responsibility of developing to their full potential is left up to them, many therapists lose their way and settle for something short of excellence.

I want to encourage you that intentional practice of your clinical reasoning and skills is one of the ways you develop your calling and reach your full potential. It takes an insatiable hunger to learn more. If you learn more and practice what you learn, you will get better. You need to be intentional with every patient you examine and treat. It is these types of intentional practices that will help you grow into an expert in a particular area of therapy. As your expertise grows, your sense of calling and preference will develop right along with your expertise.

I have one last word of warning. Professional growth demands that you are always stretching yourself outside your comfort zone. If you don't challenge yourself, you won't grow. If you keep doing only the skills that you are competent in, you won't develop as much as you could. If you are not pushing your knowledge and skill you will fail. You'll feel like you don't know what you are doing until you finally push through your unknown to develop mastery. Without a growth mentality and a willingness to put in the years of intentional practice, you won't develop mastery no matter how smart or talented you are. Your calling will become clearer to you as you fully engage in the process of challenging yourself with the guidance of wise mentors who have experienced the same process themselves.

# CALLED TO SERVE

## Brennan Hussey PT

Cash practice owner Brennan Hussey feels called to serve his community with his manual therapy skills and by coaching basketball. Brennan's father was a teacher/coach who died of a heart attack in his 50s. His father's early death had a profound impact on how Brennan was going to live his life and practice physical therapy. He determined that he wanted to live for what mattered for as long as he lived.

For Brennan that meant taking advanced training in manual therapy so that he could provide his clients the best care possible. It also meant that he would volunteer his time as a basketball coach. Being involved selflessly in his community has turned out to be his strongest marketing strategy to build his cash-based practice. Brennan has built a successful practice through deep, personal relationships with his clients, their family members and friends in his community. They know him and trust him.

The pillars of his practice are listening, taking a personal interest in his clients and a devotion to mastering his hands-on clinical effectiveness. This foundation allows him to design a profitable practice around the type of lifestyle he desires. Creating a lifestyle practice based upon his calling affords him time to do the activities he loves: Serving clients with his expertise, spending time with his family and investing in young people through coaching basketball.

**Brennan has taken a holistic view of his practice and has designed it to serve a higher purpose rather than he becoming a slave to the practice.**

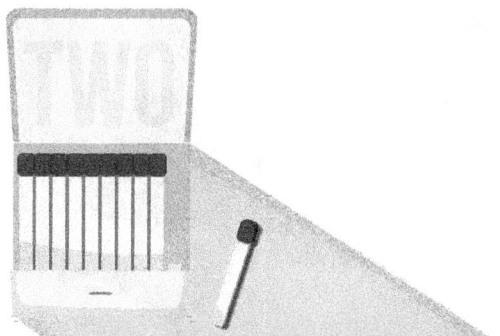

# PART TWO

# COURSE CORRECTION

*"All great changes are preceded by chaos."*
*– Deepak Chopra*

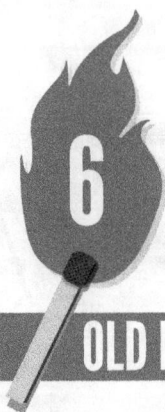

# CHAPTER SIX / OLD HEALTHCARE ECONOMY

In the U.S. therapists are in the midst of healthcare reform. Therapists bound to the old ways of providing care are struggling. In this chapter I describe three main influences impacting the delivery of therapy services.

## Cost

For several decades United States consumers, policy makers, business leaders and healthcare providers have faced recurring contradictions in trying to provide affordable healthcare in a $2.8 trillion fragmented system. Quite frankly, we have not gotten our money's worth.

Simultaneously the U.S. government is confronting a debt and deficit problem. The U.S. public debt stood at $18 trillion as of January 2015. The 2014 federal deficit was estimated at $486 Billion. But if current laws do not change, the deficit is expected to rise to about $1 trillion, mainly because of the aging population, rising healthcare costs, an expansion of federal subsidies for health insurance and growing interest payments on the federal debt.

Federal healthcare programs, primarily Medicare and Medicaid, comprise 32% of federal spending growth in the United States. Medicare is one of the largest and fastest-growing programs in the entire federal budget. Insurance coverage for a family of four will cost approximately $16,000 per year.

Obamacare, or the Affordable Care Act legislation, was signed into law in 2010 to increase the quality and affordability of health insurance. The law intends to improve coverage to the uninsured by expanding public and private insurance coverage. The Affordable Care Act's new spending is projected to cost more than $1.8 trillion dollars over the next decade. This vision of new healthcare reform can be described as a land that lies somewhere over the rainbow.

If you want to know why your professional life is changing so much in such as rapid manner you must follow the money trail. The present reimbursement system for healthcare is unsustainable. We simply cannot afford it. Government spending on entitlement programs like Medicare and Medicaid is threatening to bankrupt the country. Policy makers have had to make quick, drastic changes in order to stave off financial disaster.

To guide Congress with difficult decisions in the healthcare system, the Center for Medicare and Medicaid Services (CMS) recommends policy changes to limit spending. Constant changes in reimbursement have caused all third-party payers to examine the cost-benefit ratio of each type of healthcare service provided. Rehabilitation services are scrutinized for delivering value for the cost of that service. The over emphasis on cost has led to unintended consequences.

## Commodity

In the marketplace, transactions of goods or services are made in one of three categories: quality, value or price. In the past, most healthcare services were sold almost exclusively on quality. Government entitlement programs and insurance companies were responsible for paying the bills.

Therefore most consumers wanted the best quality healthcare available regardless of cost. The cost of healthcare is now being shifted to healthcare consumers in order to bring market forces to bear on rising costs.

Today mammoth insurance companies are paying at contracted rates with almost no regard for quality or value. Controlling rising costs is the major priority within the current reimbursement system.

The main distinction between providers is whether they are in network or out of network. Healthcare professionals are not distinguished by professional expertise or outcomes. Accessibility and convenience guide consumer choices since the price is consistent between providers.

The commoditization of rehabilitation services happens when services lose differentiation in the market. The market treats all services as equivalent with minimal regard to professional qualifications of the provider who delivered the service. This occurs when there is a dilution of the intellectual capital necessary to provide equal value to the consumer, or, in this case, the third-party payer. Value of the service is left up to market demand. The market driver is price not quality.

As third-party payers and employers shift more of the cost of medical care to the individual, the population is forced to deal with decisions on how to spend their healthcare dollars. Consumers are primed to abandon traditional methods of care for new ones that they perceive as a better value. As the healthcare industry's center of gravity shifts towards consumers, new market-savvy players are moving quickly to capitalize on this nearly $3 trillion U.S. industry.

Their services will be driven by consumer convenience and the prevention of diseases that require expensive medical intervention such as diabetes and heart disease. One example of the new competition for therapists is in the $267 billion fitness and wellness market. Personal trainers and self-proclaimed exercise specialists will aggressively compete with physical therapy services traditionally provided by highly educated professionals.

## Competition

Competition in the marketplace drives down costs. One characteristic of a commodity is that its price is determined as a function of its market as a whole. Therapists are repulsed by their services being reduced to the commodity level. Many believe in the inherent value of their service based upon the cost of their professional education and the "use value" of the person who benefits from their services. Many are oblivious to market forces and take offense when the value of their services is determined by consumers and insurance middlemen. They fail to recognize the many aspects of product or service differentiation.

Brands, the interface between the service provider and the consumer, will become increasingly important in the future. The ability to affect the perceived quality by the end user will help to set therapists' care apart from other low-cost competitors.

As healthcare policy makers and employers slowly inch towards a value-driven, pay-for-performance system, consumers may not wait for them. As deductibles and co-insurance costs rise for individuals, consumers are abandoning traditional care providers and venues for more affordable and convenient alternatives.

Many consumers who are strapped for cash will spend their own money with their most affordable option. Consumers with more disposable income will purchase healthcare services based upon quality. Others will seek value and still others will buy the cheapest alternative. The provider's degree and professional qualifications are not equally important to every type of consumer.

Traditional competitors for therapists were chiropractors and other therapists. Now therapists compete with personal trainers, yoga and pilates instructors and a variety of online fitness gurus. The axiom "if you can't beat them join them" may not be the best strategy to become a competitive player in the wellness/fitness industry. Therapists are required to maintain their professional integrity and work within the legality of their professional license.

The present healthcare system is absurdly complex and one of the most highly regulated industries in the world. Its third-party payment system is one of the biggest barriers to change. As you consider keeping your competitive edge, I encourage you to differentiate your practice by affordable value not price. While opportunities for growth are endless, they require an understanding of the consumers' needs, market realities and efficient business models.

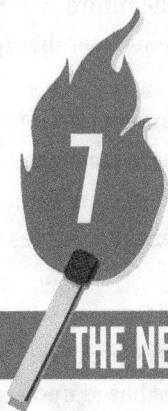

While healthcare reform through governmental legislation has often gotten the most attention, what may have escaped your notice is the giant restructuring of the economies throughout the world. This change is often referred to as the New Economy and it is drastically changing the way people work and live. Thomas Malone asks this regarding the classic "command and control" management style: "If we believe that top-down, centralized management will become less and less desirable and less and less common, the question becomes, what could take its place?" There are opportunities for businesses to step into the vacuum created by the trend towards the democratization and decentralization of healthcare services.

## Bigger isn't Better

For centuries societal success was dependent on a society's ability to create large and disciplined organizations. Stability and growth were dependent upon economies of scale and the biggest organizations, like General Electric, IBM and Ford, generally won and won big. The healthcare system followed the bigger is better model and grew from independent neighborhood doctors and hospitals run by religious orders, to massive organizations, insurance companies and government entitlement programs.

For years the U.S. spent more for healthcare on both a percentage of Gross Domestic Production and per-capita basis than any other country in the world. Spending so much on healthcare gradually hurt U.S. global competitiveness and siphoned resources away from education and infrastructure. Suddenly big wasn't better and it led to widespread dissatisfaction in the U.S. healthcare system.

Gradually society's healthcare needs changed. Large healthcare institutions were no longer able to solve national healthcare problems through immunizations and expensive emergency medicine. More people were suffering from chronic diseases associated with lifestyle rather than infectious diseases. People couldn't just take a pill to cure the heart disease or cancer that may have been brought about by choices to smoke, to eat high-calorie, high-fat food, or to live a sedentary lifestyle.

Modern medicine began to change at an accelerated pace largely due to information availability and technology. The speed of change in medicine and the healthcare economy shifted the advantages of scale to the smaller, more agile units that could change on a dime. The assumption that bigger was better wasn't always true.

This doesn't mean that large healthcare institutions will go the way of the dinosaur, but it does mean that there are now open doors for ambitious therapists to start businesses to meet consumer needs. Large organizations have many entrenched traditions and stakeholders who are anachronistic, which means that entrepreneurial-minded therapists can seize market advantage from them.

Traditionally, physicians served as the primary gatekeepers, determining a patient's primary health service needs. In the past, an insurance plan's payment was dependent upon the gatekeeper's decision of medical necessity. As the medical system shifted towards managed care and other payment mechanisms, physicians have felt their power as a gatekeeper diminish.

We live in an era of easily accessible healthcare information and people relying on any number of Internet sites for self-education when making healthcare decisions. Patients are able to do their own research, watch YouTube videos then confidently make a request to their primary care physician for a referral for the solution of their choice. The American Journal of Surgery reports that 69% of patients decided to have surgery before meeting their surgeon, and 47% stated that the surgeon did not influence their decision. I'm not saying this is better, but perhaps the trusted patient-doctor relationship has changed and maybe the gatekeeper's role as sole determiner of care has outgrown its usefulness.

## Direct Access

Direct access has been a hot topic for therapists in outpatient settings for years. Therapists are confident that their knowledge and skills can make a significant difference in people's health when they are given the chance to treat those people. Therapists talk to people every day who are unaware of exactly what they do. They listen patiently to the horror stories of failed or unnecessary surgeries, knowing that it's too late to change those situations. They wish that the system was different, allowing them to connect with the people who need their services.

Now the Internet has given therapists an opportunity to connect directly to people who need their services. The Internet has radically changed the way we live, connect and even shop. People are becoming very comfortable with buying goods and services online. According to Invesp, more than 62% of U.S. consumers with Internet access shop online at least once per month. Therapists are realizing that Millennials and the Gen Xers are shopping online for everything, and that includes physicians and therapists.

People selecting their own healthcare providers and services represents a huge shift in consumer thinking. Therapists have direct access in some form in all 50 states and patients are able to legally receive therapy services without a physician referral. Direct access to the consumer through the Internet could be the holy grail that therapists have been searching for. As deductibles rise, with some consumers having to pay as much as $10,000 in out-of-pocket expenses, people are searching online for the best value for their dollar.

Therapists are re-thinking their dependency on gatekeepers and are taking their marketing efforts online directly to consumers. Now in place of good referral sources, a therapist must have an Internet storefront—their website. Potential patients will make decisions in a matter of seconds on whether to walk into a virtual clinic or move on to the next site. A clear message of who you are and what makes you unique is critical.

## Therapy Minions?

The 2010 animated film *Despicable Me* features super villain Gru's main partners in crime, the minions. Minions are portrayed as diminutive, yellow creatures who have only one purpose in life: to serve their despicable master. Gru and his Keystone Cop minions launch a scheme to fulfill his childhood dream of being an astronaut by stealing the moon. Sometimes I wonder if we as medical professionals have become therapy minions?

Merriam-Webster defines a minion as "someone who is not powerful or important and who obeys the orders of a powerful leader or boss." In *Despicable Me* the minions are perfect sidekicks to move the story forward in a hilarious and heart-warming way. However, when a minion-like attitude is present in the new healthcare market, it's not a comedy but a tragedy.

When cost containment is the primary driving force for healthcare reform, medical care is often categorized as an expense, not as an asset. Recent trends in reimbursement for therapeutic services have shaped our perceived value in the healthcare marketplace. More tragically it has begun to refashion how we as therapists value ourselves.

In the United States, therapists, like other healthcare providers, have been reimbursed based upon volume of procedures and cost to provide those services. In essence, the more procedures you did and the more those procedures cost, the more you were paid. The fee-for-service model encouraged over utilization of services and waste by both consumers and providers. Studies estimated $700 billion was wasted on all kinds of services provided in all healthcare venues. The costs of the fee-for-service model has forced the U.S. government and insurance companies to implement fundamental changes.

The way we are reimbursed for our care will be dramatically different in the near future. The days of getting a physician to refer a steady stream of patients to your door are over. Unfortunately, I see many therapists stuck in the old economy mindset. I hear them say, "If Dr. Busy would just send more patients then my troubles would be over." We are in the midst of a transition to alternative payment models that will be value-based and pay providers according to performance. All providers, including us, will be forced to provide quality care at a lower cost. And we will have to convince the consumer that our services have value.

## Value

Value seems to be a buzzword in the field of therapy right now. Usually when therapists talk about their value they often equate it to the cost of their education and experience. Their thinking goes like this: To become a therapist I traded something of value, money, often a great deal of money, and six or seven years out of my life in exchange for a professional degree. The exchange of something of significant worth to me makes my time worth an equally significant wage or hourly. Most therapists have little understanding of economics and the healthcare market. They really have no realistic idea of the value they deliver to customers, and most are ill prepared to quantify their unique value in order to help them stand out in the market place. The third-party payer system is partly to blame for insulating therapists from the supply and demand forces that drive other industries. Your ability to identify and defend the value of your services has become vital to your business survival.

Therapists often confuse the value of our services with our professional assets—our training, expertise and therapeutic skill. We often describe the features and scientific basis of our offerings in terms that no one but other therapists can understand. Instead, we should tell of the benefits that the consumer receives from our professional care. Facts about this or that technique or program do not mean nearly as much to consumers as an explanation about the benefits they will receive and how therapy can save them money in the long run.

In the simplest of terms, value is the clear and quantified benefit your unique services provide to the consumer along with the financial impact. If you are like most therapists, you have no clear, unique value proposition to present to your potential customers. That must change.

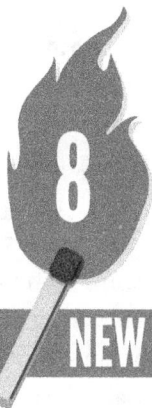

# CHAPTER EIGHT / NEW CONSUMERS

There is a new buyer in town, a buyer who wants to know the value she is getting for her dollar. This buyer might be your patient or a third-party payer. In either case she wants a clear explanation of the costs and benefits of your services before she hands over any money.

This buyer is also impatient. The U.S. healthcare system, while it often provides life-saving interventions and medical miracles, has completely failed to create an efficient business model to deliver affordable routine care, and buyers have moved on. As healthcare reform makes glacial progress towards a consumer-centered future, buyers are racing ahead looking for innovative companies and individuals to satisfy their healthcare demand now.

And they are looking in alternative places. New players, from retail, technology, telecommunications, consumer products and trusted brands, are shaping consumer expectations and purchasing habits. Over time these new players will siphon off billions of dollars from traditional healthcare systems while expanding the less regulated fitness and wellness market.

Similar to other U.S. industries like banking, entertainment and retail, consumers are becoming more comfortable in abandoning traditional healthcare providers. A new survey by Price Waterhouse Coopers Health

Research Institute found that consumers are willing to abandon traditional care venues for more affordable and convenient alternatives. Nearly one in two respondents said they would choose new options for more than a dozen common medical procedures.

Companies like CVS and Wal-Mart intend to expand aggressively into not only the pharmacy market but also into other healthcare products and services. The CVS Minute Clinic started in 2000 and is the leading retail medical clinic in the United States. It has provided care through 24 million patient visits.

Healthcare provided by retail giants will shift consumer expectations and decentralize care away from traditional organizations like hospitals and therapy clinics. Consumers will be able to access care with greater convenience and less cost. Therapy clinics will face critical decisions on how to compete for the disposable income spent by young families. Will they chase commodity-driven revenue or develop premium services that deliver unique value on a personal basis?

The shift also means new types of career opportunities for courageous therapists. In his article "The High-Res Society," Paul Graham writes: "Large organizations will start to do worse now, though, because for the first time in history they're no longer getting the best people. An ambitious kid graduating from college now doesn't want to work for a big company. They want to work for the hot startup that's rapidly growing into one. If they're really ambitious, they want to start it."

Bright, ambitious therapists no longer content to climb the corporate ladder are launching startups and building their ladders as they go. These therapists start with consumers' needs and desires and work backwards. They let undistracted focus on satisfying the buyer guide their creation of services, operations, location and hours.

Opportunities abound for smart, courageous therapists. Those who are wise will read the market and capitalize on strategic options. Some of the best opportunities might lie in serving buyers who are looking for ways to maintain function and independence as they age.

## Boomer Geriatrics

Baby Boomers grew up listening to Elvis and the Beatles, drove fast cars, and took political and social protests to the streets. They were born between 1946 and 1964. The 78 million U.S. Baby Boomers have influenced cultural trends, lifestyles and social institutions. As the Baby Boomers age they are going to have a tremendous impact on American healthcare for years to come. If you are a therapist considering owning your own practice, they are a demographic you can't afford to ignore.

Consider this: By the year 2020, approximately one billion people will be over the age of 60. Another one million will turn 65 every week. By 2017 one out of two people will be over the age of 50. These numbers point to a significant demographic shift. Baby Boomers are going to be responsible for a significant portion of all healthcare dollars spent for several decades to come. I hear many ambitious young therapists say they only want to work with athletes and manual therapy. Good luck with that. Those are two of the most competitive therapy specializations. Sports medicine is a narrow niche in a crowded market with limited resources. In contrast, let's look at the economic impact of Baby Boomers.

On average an adult over the age of 50 spends one out of every two dollars spent in the United States. By 2017, older adults will spend seven out of ten disposable dollars. That's 7.1 trillion spent annually comprises 46% of the gross domestic product in the United States.

Older people spend more of their income on health than anything else. Boomers also expect much more for their money than their parents did. The influx and demands of older adults have forced the healthcare industry to change its ways or be left behind. You, too, will miss out if your services aren't Boomer friendly. Wellness and health promotion services are in demand as Boomers experience the physiological effects of aging. Boomers will seek out trusted experts who will help them age successfully. Plus they have the cash to pay for it. You can hardly afford to miss out on the opportunity to serve older adults with your much needed therapy skills. If you are still interested only in working with athletes, you will find an abundance of older athletes who will gladly pay for your expertise.

## Successful Aging

Physical activity is the foundation for successful aging. Boomers want professional assistance as they manage changes in functional abilities, strength, balance and cardiovascular capacity. As Boomers try to maintain their maximum quality of life and independence, they will need wellness Sherpas. Therapists are perfectly equipped and experienced to guide Boomers as they navigate the mountain of successful aging. The ability to understand the needs of Boomers from their point of view is critical. If you practice ageism, even unknowingly, older adults will pick up on your prejudicial attitude and go somewhere else. If you design your services with a cultural sensitivity towards older adults, they will beat down your doors to work with you.

## Aging in Place

There is a strong movement in the U.S. towards assisting older adults to successfully age while remaining in their own homes. The home is where older adults desire to live and is by far the most cost-effective option. To remain independent at home usually requires a strong physical capacity. Currently, only one third of Americans age 65 and older are completely able to take care of themselves and be independent in their daily activities.

There is a normal gradual decline in functional abilities as people age. The healthcare system typically acts as a safety net to rehabilitate people if they drop below a certain disability threshold. When a person becomes unable to independently perform their daily activities, resources are usually made available. In comparison, minimal resources are invested in non-disabled individuals to help them maintain or enhance independence and prevent disability.

Assisting older adults to age in place is a magnificent opportunity to contribute to our society's wellbeing. Functional independence, either physical or cognitive, is less about chronological age and more about functional age. Many older adults are at high risk of losing their independence and ability to age at home. Frail seniors are at high risk for falls and broken bones, events which frequently act as the entry into institutional care.

Therapists must go beyond the current medical model to deliver a broad range of programs that focus on wellness and prevention. Fall prevention, home safety assessments, and virtual Internet fitness programs are examples of creative solutions. And with more patients wanting end-of-life care at home, therapists can partner with palliative care and hospice teams. Older adults and their children are searching for professional in-home services. Perhaps your business model can include fitness and prevention services delivered to older adults on a cash basis.

# DOOR TO DOOR

## Karen Litzy PT

### "I walk to my patients homes to treat them."

Karen Litzy is the creator of an independent home-based therapy practice in New York City. She uses the public transportation system to provide private in-home healthcare and personal training services throughout the city. She is an excellent example of a therapist who has created a way to follow her heart in a unique and unconventional manner.

Karen gradually started her own cash-based business over the course of eight years. She developed her clientele as a full-time personal trainer at several clubs, then offered a more convenient service by going to where her clients lived and worked. By offering services beyond the clinic walls she's able to keep overhead low and personalized service high. Karen grew an extensive network of referral sources from satisfied patients and physicians. She has also cultivated a solid working relationship with trainers, massage therapists and alternative medicine professionals.

Karen connects with other cash-based therapists throughout the country through interviews on her podcast Healthy, Wealthy and Smart. She builds her online brand by educating her followers on how to live a happy, healthy, pain-free life.

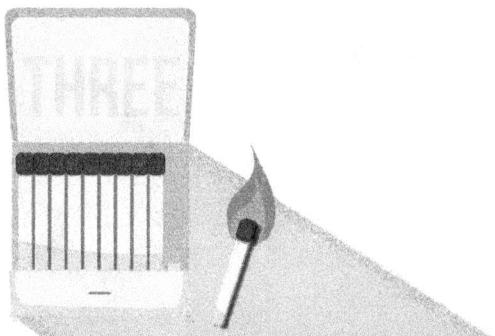

# THREE

# PART THREE

## COURSE OF ACTION

*"I shall be telling this with a sigh*
*Somewhere ages and ages hence:*
*Two roads diverged in a wood, and I–*
*I took the one less traveled by,*
*And that has made all the difference."*
*–Robert Frost*

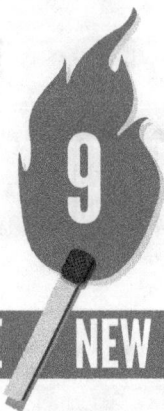

# CHAPTER NINE / NEW PRACTICE MODEL

A growing number of healthcare providers are opting out of the third-party payer system and have switched to a cash-based practice. This emerging business model goes by a variety of names: cash-based, cash-only, concierge-based, membership-based or out-of-network practice are a few. Therapy practices most often identify themselves as cash-based or out-of-network. Whatever the name, these self-identified therapists have opted out of the insurance system almost completely.

This is an important distinction to make. For decades there have been hybrid clinics that have offered cash-only wellness services in addition to the traditional insurance-based therapy. Medical fitness centers have expanded all over the country and offer fitness and wellness services such as cardiac rehab, yoga, personal training, medical spa, massage, pool programs and group fitness classes. The owners range from mom-and-pop private practices with an integrated fitness center to large hospital and retirement communities offering elaborate facilities, staff and programs.

The cash-based therapy model I am describing is a small therapy practice of one or two owners that has made the leap to opt out of the insurance system completely. The primary reason for choosing this model is one word: Freedom.

## Personal Freedom

Therapists who only accept cash payment are freed from the burden of insurance regulations and paperwork. They are able to have longer treatment times to achieve the desired outcomes for their patients. Better outcomes lead to improved client and therapist satisfaction.

## Professional Freedom

Third-party reimbursement rules often dictate how therapists treat their clients. Therapists feel pressure to utilize certain procedures based upon reimbursement rather than evidence of effectiveness. Decreased reimbursements have contributed to pressure on therapists to meet productivity quotas that compete with standards of quality. Therapists in a cash-based model have freedom to treat clients according to the latest evidence, and to work with clients suited to their expertise.

## Financial Freedom

The fee-for-service model doesn't necessarily reward healthcare providers for getting patients better in a cost-effective manner. However, in a cash-based practice, cost-conscious, expert therapists are rewarded directly by the consumer for the quality, effective care they deliver.

Clinics that accept insurance reimbursement often have larger staffs in order to administer the claims process. The higher personnel costs— often as much as 60% of revenue—means these therapists must see more patients and complete more paperwork. All of this takes time away from direct patient care. Therapists who have adopted a cash-only business model get paid for the value they deliver to their clients. The economics are straightforward. If you don't deliver value consistently by helping clients achieve their health goals, you don't grow your business. Therapists often feel a sense of reward for being accountable for the results they deliver.

Many therapists are experiencing success with cash-based practices. They have bet their careers that they could achieve financial success AND pursue their passions. As they do, they find they are more creative and effective. They are also respected for their expertise and hard work.

# ADVANTAGES OF CASH-BASED THERAPY PRACTICE

## Personal Connection with Clients

The new healthcare economy allows cash-based therapists to have direct access. Yes, that's right, the same direct access that therapists have been striving for legislatively all these years. The shift in economics and the Internet has provided a direct connection to potential clients.

You don't have to play by the rules of the old economy anymore. Below the surface you can find countless examples in other industries that are bypassing traditional gatekeepers. In the music and book publishing industries, artists and authors are gate jumping by using social media and distribution channels like iTunes and Amazon.com to market directly to their fans. Therapists are starting to the do the same.

Earlier I introduced Aaron LeBauer of lebauerpt.com. Aaron had established a successful massage therapy practice prior to getting his physical therapy degree. As a therapist he developed a primary care mindset. This mindset freed him to bypass the physician gatekeeper to focus on the needs of his patients. Aaron overcame the fear of upsetting the doctor by focusing on delivering what his clients wanted in the first place—great value.

All around us the physician gatekeepers of the old healthcare system are becoming impotent. As gatekeepers, they are faced with increased competition and pressure to hold down costs. Large hospitals and Physician-Owned Physical Therapy Services (POPTS) control the clinical pathways and direct patients into their own organizations to maintain profitability. Therapists bound to the old physician-referral system are facing serious competition for those precious declining referrals.

New media opportunities have leveled the playing field. You can gain an edge by marketing your services directly to your ideal clients through social media. Prospective patients can easily access you and learn about you and your services. The bad news for gatekeepers is that patients are coming into their offices empowered with information and power to inform the gatekeeper of their choice of providers. The referral is becoming less autocratic and more democratized. Direct access through the Internet allows you to develop a meaningful connection to a potential patient prior to their surgery or visit to the physician.

## Value Connection with Clients

Therapists in a cash-based practice must be willing to put their skills and their value to the test to make money. The marketplace is the ultimate determiner of the value of your services. When therapists have their own "skin in the game," there is a concentration on the essentials and on what really is valuable in the eyes of the consumer.

Instead of trying to be good at everything, cash-based therapists focus on their strengths, develop unique value and work hard to grow their practices. Even if you don't end up owning your own clinic or working for yourself, it would benefit you to get to know the consumers and develop your expertise, then fill your schedule with ideal clients who will benefit from that expertise.

There is not a practice niche that is too crowded for innovation and fresh thinking. The therapists who are in tune with their clients' needs have a tremendous advantage over traditional big business. Therapists with the freedom to infuse professional expertise with a fresh approach will always be in demand and ahead of the curve. Therapists who combine their talent with solid branding and direct marketing to consumers have the foundation to build a thriving consumer-centric business.

## Job Security

I know it seems counter intuitive but I want to challenge the notion that a large corporation is the safest place for a good therapy job. Therapists have enjoyed a long run of growing demand for their services. Projections of our aging population indicate that demand will extend for at least a few more decades. The question is not what the future job market is, but what the future job description for therapists will be.

One of the reasons that therapists worked for big organizations in the old healthcare economy was job security. Therapists could count on a steady stream of referrals, treat patients, toe the company line and they'd be good for a 30- to 40-year career. With corporate mergers and government entitlement programs being scrutinized, therapists can no longer assume that their future is safe with large corporate employers. More importantly, the quality of their professional life may not contribute to the type of work-life fulfillment they dreamed of.

I realize that traditional employment will to be how most therapists earn a living. There is a certain comfort to this employment option. However, therapists should not assume that these employment situations are the ideal way to advance their professional career.

All of us can learn from entrepreneurial therapists on how to take smart professional risks, and how to fight for quality patient care and against corporate greed or ignorance. I personally found less risk and more reward by steering my career toward working for myself. The compromises I might have been asked to make by a large hospital would have stifled my dreams and drained my soul. If you want to steer your own ship, the following chapters will help you navigate your journey. In the next section I outline the steps to build your dream practice and take control of your career.

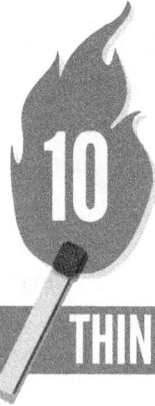

# CHAPTER TEN / THINK TRIATHLON

Starting and managing your own therapy practice is like completing in a triathlon. Unlike a marathon or a bike race, a triathlon presents a unique challenge to even the fittest of athletes. A triathlete must complete three separate but continuous endurance disciplines. The most popular types of triathlons include swimming, biking and running. The total time of all three events counts toward how well you perform. You can be a great swimmer but a lousy runner and not do well. Or you could be the fastest biker but sink like a rock in the water and not be competitive. Elite triathletes pride themselves in being total athletes, as evidenced by their by their competitive performance in multiple events.

You might think of starting a cash-based therapy practice as your own Iron Man triathlon. Your three events are:

## 1. Clinical Expertise
## 2. Marketing Expertise
## 3. Business Expertise

Creating value through your therapy skill is only one event in a successful cash-based practice. The other equally important areas of expertise are marketing and business. You could be a world famous expert but if no one knows about you, your practice will languish in obscurity. Your schedule could be packed because you're in such high demand that you have to turn people away. But if you don't know your cost of treatment or have a handle on cash flow, you could end up a slave to your new business.

## Clinical Expert

Your practice will be built upon what you are good at and what people want. A successful practice will meet the needs of your ideal clients. You need to become known as a trusted expert who solves people's problems. You need to develop expertise in relieving your patients' pain and/or helping them to reach their health goals. Your client exchanges something of value, e.g. money, time, effort, for benefit. You deliver what your client values, pain relief, better performance or improved quality of life.

Therapists who are successful in a cash therapy practice are typically highly skilled with a concentrated area of expertise. They have a solid professional therapeutic foundation and experience. However, they almost always have a unique skill or service through which they stand out from the competition. They do not try to be all things to all people, but to be an expert to a few.

Therapists often struggle early on when establishing their therapy brand. They underestimate their professional training and experience. In addition, they take for granted the expertise and the people skills they've developed as a good therapist. It's just what they do. It's part of the job.

So many times therapists don't see their own assets because they are trying so hard to be like someone else. The key to discovering your own worth is to spend less time looking outward and more time looking inward.

Ask yourself the following questions: Who am I? What are my greatest talents or gifts? Do I have any special abilities or unique experiences that give me an edge? Am I an expert in a field of study or special technique? Listen to what previous clients and friends say about you. How do they consistently describe you to others?

While you are doing this exercise in self-examination you might find it beneficial to make a distinction between your personal assets and your professional assets. It's easy to confuse your personal value with your market value. You turn your professional assets into a service or product that you sell to the market. Just remember, the market determines the value of your service. Your focus is to be yourself and package your service in a way that your ideal client will pay for it.

## Marketing Expert

Let's be honest here, what comes to mind when you hear the word marketing? Typically therapists will say things like pushy, sleazy, annoying, aggressive, difficult, scary. So before we get too far into this area I'd like to develop a working definition of marketing, or else you'll never develop the mindset to attract and keep new clients.

The dictionary defines marketing as the action or business of promoting and selling products or services, including market research and advertising. That stuffy definition is out of date and not at all useful for therapists who want to connect with clients. Let's toss that out and go with something like this: Marketing is taking action to build helpful, long-term connections with people.

I think that most therapists already have basic skills in marketing. They just don't know it. Today's consumer is bombarded daily with thousands of marketing messages and they have learned to tune them out. Consumers are seeking trusted experts who can help them with their problems. You can be that trusted expert.

Marketing isn't cheesy salesman tactics. It isn't pushy self-promotion that makes you uncomfortable. Marketing is learning how to reach out and maintain long-term connections with people and using your knowledge and skill to make their lives healthier. It's as simple as that.

Now we'll look at the type of people you will want to connect when marketing your practice.

## Loyal Fans

Customer lifetime value (CLV) is a marketing term you should be acquainted with. Customer lifetime value is simply a prediction of all the value your business can expect to receive from your entire connection with a customer. A simple CLV analysis would take into account factors like average revenue earned with each purchase, frequency of purchase, length of time between purchases and acquisition costs.

Improving your CLV can have a dramatic impact of the success of your business. In the simplest terms, repeat appointments from satisfied clients is where you will make your profit.

The Pareto Principle is worth mentioning here. The Pareto Principle simply states that for a variety of situations, approximately 80% of results will come from 20% of the causes. When you apply it to a cash-based clinic, it means that 80% of your revenue will be generated from 20% of your clients. Whether the percentages are exact is not the point. The principle generally is true that some of your customers are worth a whole lot more than others. Identifying and staying connected to your ideal clients is extremely valuable to your business.

## Business Expert

Assess your strengths and aptitude towards marketing and running a business. Be determined to learn the basic principles in both areas. You can put in the effort required to learn and grow in your weaker areas, or you can decide to get help from someone else.

Technology has made running a company on a smaller scale more economical and effective. Many entrepreneurs are leveraging technology to compete with larger companies at a fraction of the cost. The game changers have found the Internet to be an invaluable resource for timely learning opportunities, topic-specific books and the ability to make valuable connections with other therapists via social media to learn the most effective path to success.

Much of the rest of the book is about business expertise as it relates to the four stages of business development.

# LEARN FROM EXPERTS

## Jarod Carter PT, DPT, MTC

Jarod Carter is considered by many to be the front-runner in the cash-based physical therapy movement. Jarod began Carter Physiotherapy in April 2010 as a cash-only private practice.

Jarod graduated from University of St. Augustine PT School in 2005. He developed his clinical expertise further by earning certifications in Manual Therapy and CSCS. Throughout his young career he purposely sought out employment opportunities where manual therapists and business experts could mentor him.

He thoughtfully went into business for himself by diving right into a cash-based solo practice. He soon developed a reputation for getting incredibly fast results through one-hour sessions of one-on-one care. Creative marketing combined with solid business principles led to him being booked solid within six months.

At his website, DrJarodCarter.com, Jarod is paying it forward by helping other therapists to start their own cash-based practices. Through his podcast, blog and books he is providing the latest information on private pay physical therapy services.

**He is an online mentor to many entrepreneurs who dream of spending more time with patients by owning their own cash-based therapy practice.**

# DREAM PRACTICE ROAD MAP:

## Four Essential Stages for Business Success

By now many of you are convinced that the cash-based therapy practice is worth considering. Some of you may have thought about owning your own practice for some time but you don't know where to start. The next section will help you to understand the stages that I think your business should go through. I've worked with and learned from many successful business owners over my 35-year career. I've combined business principles from the past with new entrepreneurial strategies found in great books like *The Lean Startup* by Eric Ries, *Book Yourself Solid* by Michael Port and *Platform* by Michael Hyatt. I've written down my insights on what you will most likely experience when starting your small business. It is a roadmap to guide your journey towards owning your own practice.

Let me confess that I'm envious of you. I wish I'd had this sort of roadmap when I started my practice way back when. Having a guide for achieving my dreams would have helped me to be more focused and to reach my goals sooner. As you take steps toward owning your own practice, the more motivated and confident you'll become. Going through the four stages I recommend will help you avoid costly mistakes and feel less overwhelmed. Understanding how businesses are built and whom you are called to serve will set you up for success as you define it.

You won't necessarily go through all the stages in sequence. You might find yourself working in a couple of stages at once. You may go back to clarify a previous stage once you've gained practical experience. It is a major mistake to think that there is one route to a successful cash-based practice. There are as many routes as there are therapists with unique dreams and skills. Feel free to experiment and discover your own path to your dream destination. I hope my evolving road map will help you from spinning your wheels and getting stuck in a dead end.

Before we look at the road map to own your practice I want you to understand something. A career journey is much more than a trip. A trip is when you travel somewhere, share experiences, take pictures and come back home. A journey could be defined as a quest to get you from point A to point B. If you decide to travel down the road to your dream practice, you do it without plans to return. You'll change along the way. Your journey will have all the excitement, drama, hardships and adventures of the *Lord of the Rings*. It involves both leaving what's behind and pressing forward with persistence. There will be nothing boring about it, and it will require your best efforts. I invite you to take the next step in your life's journey.

## Dream Practice Road Map

I'm going to walk you through the four stages of business growth, point out road signs to look for and dead-ends to avoid. Let's get started. The four stages that I believe every practice will go through are:

## Stage One: Set Up
## Stage Two: Start Up
## Stage Three: Step Up
## Stage Four: Stand Out

Many of you will want the step-by-step details to assist you in starting up your own business. Detailed information on how to start and manage a successful practice is beyond the scope of this book. In the future I will release practical resources to help you grow your dream practice. I will incorporate input from readers and the latest trends into additional material. You'll find new resources on my website at paulpotterpt.com.

Think of the practice road map as the 30,000-foot view to help you get perspective and determine your starting point. Knowing your location and having a sense of direction can make the difference between developing a successful business and wasting a whole lot of time and money.

## Stage One: Set Up

The Set-Up stage is about design. You'll want to design a practice based upon your unique calling and business realities. The goal of this stage is for you to understand how a business is built and whom you will serve. Before you take steps towards any destination you'll need to prepare. You'll want to research your journey's end and make a packing list of what you'll need for success. A backpack contains only the essentials that you take on your journey. It has different compartments and limited space. You have to make decisions on what you are going to take and what you are going to leave. In order to make these choices you'll need to explore a few key areas. Looking at your calling, expectations and niche helps you to define your practice and your ideal clients. In this stage you'll begin to draft a brief business plan around your calling. You'll begin to map out a route that makes sense.

## Road Signs of Stage One: Calling & Connection

I feel strongly that each of us was designed for a specific calling while on earth. You will be at your best and be the most fulfilled when you are living out that calling. You are not here to help everyone, but you are uniquely gifted to serve a specific few. Spend time to discover your calling and your unique audience.

As you investigate your possibilities, it is critical that you make meaningful connections. You'll want to have in-depth conversations with previous patients and potential clients. Active listening and asking good questions will help you extract ideas to enable you to solve their problems and ease their pain. Interview potential customers before you construct anything. Begin to narrow down what problem you are going to solve for them. Research how others are approaching the same problem. Competition isn't necessarily bad. It means there is a market for your idea and you'll just have to define your unique approach.

You will also want to connect with other therapists who have been successful in a cash-based practice. Listening to pioneers who are flourishing in their niche will help you to formulate your own practice emphasis. Social media has made connecting with industry experts easier than ever. You can join conversations on Twitter, Facebook and LinkedIn forums. Successful role models will help you narrow the possibilities as you clarify your own path.

## Dead Ends of Stage One: Compulsion & Comparison

You can waste days and months in the planning stage without making a decision and moving forward. You never actually start on your journey because you are stuck in preparation. You can squander hours naming your business, designing a logo or writing a business plan. It seems like you are making progress but you're not taking action on the things that truly matter. Initiating conversations with strangers can be intimidating, but overcoming self-doubts and risks with courageous action is what fulfilling your calling is all about. You might as well get used to it.

Making connections with successful role models can also be intimidating. You can easily get stuck comparing yourself to therapists who seem to have it all together. It is sometimes hard for leaders to remember what it was like when they were at the beginning stage. Instead of getting down on yourself, try to use their success as an inspiration. Try to pick up on early lessons learned as you stay in your own lane and make steady progress. It's a big mistake to stay in your own head and go it alone. You'll want to interview potential customers and experts before you build anything.

## Stage Two: Start Up

The Start-Up stage is about testing the waters. You'll need to embrace learning by doing. You are going to make mistakes in this phase but that's okay. It's through trial and error that you will discover the desires, dreams and personal struggles of your ideal clients. You'll need patience, persistence and lots of hustle to keep going. The start-up phase can be unpredictable and messy. It is often not a straight and well-lit path. Part of the messiness of this stage is that in addition to starting up your business you most likely are working a full-time or a couple of part-time jobs.

Early in this stage you will name your business, set goals and develop a workflow to achieve those goals. You will set up your business legally and financially. You will build your website, design a logo and business cards all meant to communicate what you see as your unique calling in the therapy field. It will begin to feel real. It is in this stage that you will develop discipline and habits to get the things done that matter the most.

Since you are the primary source of energy and income, you will be the main producer. You are building your client list. You are networking. You are treating clients. You are hustling to get things done. You are beginning to develop a critical understanding of your clients' needs and how to deliver value. You are learning under fire but you are learning how to set priorities.

## Road Signs of Stage Two: Keep it Simple

During the start-up phase you are learning what works without spreading yourself too thin. You are testing out your ideas and processes. You are beginning to develop a viable group of ideal clients who know you, trust you and are willing to pay. The key is not to deliver too many services at one time or to try to help everyone. You'll begin to know who is your ideal client and what they are looking for. You'll experiment online and offline to find out where and when clients look for professional help.

You may need to do some work for free to gain experience and to get in front of your clients. Look for opportunities to be generous with your knowledge, especially speaking in front of groups. Other sources of income provide flexibility to explore and learn while you refine your service and business. Keep your approach simple and don't move too quickly. It's wise to take your time, learn as you go and build your practice over time. When you find your sweet spot you will be at your best and people will pay you for the value you deliver.

## Dead Ends of Stage Two: Self-Doubt

At this stage your expectations and calling play a big part in your growth. Self-doubt will whisper that you don't have what it takes. It will tell you that you that you are too young, too old, too inexperienced, that you aren't skilled enough or that you aren't worth what you charge. The temptation is to throw in the towel and go back to your previous therapy job if you can.

The only way to fight off this inner voice is to remember why you decided to start your business in the first place. It is your sense of calling that will pull you through the resistance and challenges. You will need to tap into the strength of your calling and remember that there are people who need you—people you are uniquely gifted to serve.

## Stage Three: Step Up

This is the stage where you are consistently making a profit. At last all your hard work and persistence is starting to pay off. It's a great feeling. It is awesome doing the work you love, having clients who appreciate your work and being paid fairly. At the same time you may still have another job on the side to make ends meet. You begin to wonder if you can step it up and do this full time.

A lot of growth needs to happen in this stage to produce a steady source of income. You'll face several important decisions and you'll want to make those decisions based upon reliable information. To determine the viability of your practice you'll need reliable metrics. Tracking the right business numbers is essential for long-term sustainability. You have been gathering and analyzing customer feedback and sales data all along in the previous stages. Key metrics will help you determine if you are going to bootstrap your practice or borrow money. You will analyze your fees against the cost of treatment. Your metrics will help you determine if you need to pivot your business, adapt your practice or add offerings to your core professional services.

In this stage you explore different services based upon lots of ongoing conversations with ideal clients. You evolve your uniquely valuable service by improving or reducing features. You experiment with different options to find the service/market fit that feels right to you. You strengthen connections with other professionals who are regularly referring clients to you. You begin to feel the strain of running the whole business and begin to think about hiring someone or adding a partner.

The main focus of this stage is to grow your revenue to a previously determined number that will sustain your personal and professional livelihood. You may have to repeat your analysis for several months or years depending upon the market and your ideal number.

## Road Signs of Stage Three: Less but Better

Working hard is important, but more effort does not automatically mean more results. I encourage you to adopt a less-but-better approach to your practice. You may have a hard time getting comfortable with the less-but-better concept, especially if working more has paid off for you in the past. When we have been rewarded for doing more, we fall into the trap of doing more and more and more. Yet at a certain point for all of us, doing more leads to a plateau in our growth, and possibly a dip.

During this stage you need say no to many good opportunities in order to pursue the truly great ones.

If you want to grow your business, you will have to embrace tradeoffs. By definition saying yes to the best opportunity requires saying no to others. As painful as it can be, forcing yourself to analyze your options and choose your best strategy will significantly increase the likelihood of a successful outcome. Instead of thinking about "What am I giving up?" focus on "What am I going big on?" This one subtle change in your thinking can have a far-reaching effect on your life and business.

## Dead Ends of Stage Three: No Space

Entrepreneurs are movers and shakers. Usually during the step-up phase they are on the go from morning until night, day after day. There is a danger at this stage to never slow down, to fall into the trap of trying to do it all. Instead of choosing one option, you'll try to do both. Everything starts to blur together and it becomes difficult to distinguish the important from the inconsequential. It is very tempting to react to the latest trend or jump on the bandwagon of the newest business success if you don't take time to think. It is critical in this stage to create space to breathe and take time to think. In order to innovate and grow you need a way to escape the noise.

In our time-hungry society you'll need to regularly create space in your schedule to look back, look inside and look forward. Uninterrupted space enables you to reflect upon client feedback, explore different options and look at the big picture.

It is important in the growth phase to stop moving and to analyze your practice metrics. Confront yourself with the numbers that tell you what is really working and what is not. Space allows you to think about your calling and your long-term vision. It gives you permission to examine your actions to see if you are heading in the direction you want to go. There will be many course corrections and iterations along your journey. Taking time to regularly assess your progress and your direction is key to enjoying the journey.

## Stage Four: Stand Out

Even though you never stop growing your business, this stage is where you have freedom to think about other opportunities. You enjoy more financial and creative freedom than you've ever had before. In this phase you work more on your business rather than just in your business. You've transitioned into more of a CEO mode as you've hired people and are leading a team. You provide your team with a vision and the resources to do their jobs well. Your personal and company operating systems are more efficient. Your clients respect and enjoy working with you. They are eager to recommend your services to their friends and family. The majority of your clients probably come to you through word-of-mouth. The referrers that believe in you have created a snowball effect that builds over time. You've refined your pricing model based upon the value of the benefits you provide. You are comfortable selling because of the trust and credibility you have established in the community. You find your schedule is booked solid for weeks in advance.

This is another decision point in your business. It's when you decide to grow or to scale back and keep it simple. More isn't always better and it may not be what you truly want. Many business owners are choosing a business model that accommodates a desired lifestyle. They are prioritizing families, health and other personal values then building a business that fits those priorities.

To expand your business you will need to decide whether you are going to find a business partner, borrow money, or hire someone to run the operation. As you optimize your business model and build your team you'll begin to experience freedom like you've never had before. You'll enjoy the fruit of all your hard work in the previous stages by taking time off and having the business excel without you.

## Road Signs of Stage Four: Follow Your Calling

Reaching this stage of your business can feel like you are standing on a mountaintop, but it's not the end of the journey. When your business is enjoying financial stability it is important to stay true to your calling. With no clear vision or purpose, therapists may pursue projects that achieve short-term benefits. Sometimes there is little awareness of how these momentary gains advance or distract from the long-term mission. Being intentional about your purpose will help you answer the question, "How will I know when we've succeeded?" A true calling guides your sense of purpose and helps you map out the path for your business and your life.

As your profits grow and you become more organized, it is important that you build a team. You will need to be able to clearly articulate your vision so that you can attract people who share your calling. You need people on your team who understand the long-term goals of your practice and are committed to helping you get there.

## Dead Ends of Stage Four: Burnout

One of the cul-de-sacs of this stage is relying on the habits and strategies that helped your success in the previous stages. It is essential that you break out of the super hero mindset. This stage is where you learn how to delegate, organize and design systems so your business runs smoothly.

Most of us start up our practices as a one-person show. You may have the drive and energy to work 14-hour days but afterwards you crash. Since money was tight you may have developed the habit of doing most tasks yourself.

We manage the practice mostly within our own heads. As your practice grows you'll find yourself thinking about it all the time. Eventually this catches up with you and your dream practice will leave you stressed, overworked and not any good to anyone, including your family. As the practice grows you'll need to hire staff to handle client satisfaction, tech support and outreach. Outsourcing these responsibilities will leave you free to optimize your business in other ways. Organizing, delegating and eliminating are what it takes to transition from a one-person start up into a thriving business. When you as the owner choose to build a team rather than burn out, then you have made the final step in building a successful practice.

## Where Do You Go From Here?

As far as I'm concerned the writing is on the wall. Our healthcare economy has drastically changed directions and is not turning back. Yesterday's institutions (governments, universities, large corporations) that were counted on to provide career stability are wavering. Generations of therapists worked decades sheltered by stable healthcare institutions. All a therapist had to do was get on the career highway, set cruise control and take the right exit towards retirement. Now those highways may lead to nowhere and there is mass confusion about where to turn. If you've lost your professional sense of direction you, are not alone.

The main issue I see for therapists today is risk. More financial risk has been transferred to healthcare providers in the form of productivity demands, big data performance standards and lean workplace practices. In exchange for our hard work, loyalty and keeping the rules, big hospitals and corporations used to shelter us from risk. I can assure you that belief in such protection is now a fantasy. The riskiest thing you could do is to hold up your end of the bargain with the hope that the corporations will respond in kind.

The reality is that in the new healthcare economy we are all entrepreneurs. The sooner you adopt an entrepreneurial mindset the better you'll be equipped to thrive in the rapidly changing marketplace. Cash-based therapy owners have lived with risk as a fact of life and have learned to adapt to the market. As healthcare continues to change, therapists who have learned to manage risk will rise to the top. Now is the time to act.

Most people who read this book, regrettably, may resolve to take charge of their circumstances and then do nothing about it. When faced with the challenge of change, it is understandable to want to retreat to a safe harbor of good intentions. But now is not a time for good intentions. If you want to live out your calling and stay true to your professional and ethical values, you'll need more than good intentions.

On a practical level, you are most likely to need a new education in small business management and online marketing, including social media, technologies and branding. Fortunately, there are an abundance of excellent websites that provide online courses and free resources. You can get the practical training you need within the comfort of your own home without having to get your MBA.

At my website, PaulPotterPT.com, I'm building a community of therapists who want to help each other take control of their careers. I've packed a lot of information into these pages. To help you put this information into practice, I've created checklists, worksheets and other free resources. You can download them now at www.PaulPotterPT.com/cash-therapy-practice.

I suggest you get started right away. Most of it you'll learn by doing. The sooner you begin your journey the faster you'll grow your therapy platform and the more connections you'll make.

After you finish this book, put it down and get on the Internet. Find a group of therapists who share your calling and interests. Whatever your practice interest you'll find like-minded therapists out there who share your passion and will help you in practical ways to make a living doing what you love. They will be your support group who will travel the journey beside you.

There has never been a better time to create your own practice and make it successful. A practice that gives you personal and professional freedom while doing the work you love. But now—right now—is the time to take action. The choice is yours.

# Notes

1. Carol S. Dweck, Ph.D., *Mindset: The New Psychology of Success* (New York: Ballantine Books, 2006).

2. Stephen R. Covey, *Seven Habits of Highly Effective People: Powerful Lessons in Personal Change* (New York: Simon & Schuster 2004).

3. Aaron LeBauer DPT, LeBauer Consulting, http://www.lebauerconsulting.com.

4. Malcolm Gladwell, *Tipping Point: How Little Things Can Make a Difference* (Little, Brown and Company, 2000).

5. Ed Payne, "Report: Healthcare Website Failed Test Ahead of Rollout", http://www.cnn.com, October 2013.

6. Richard Piersol, "CoOportunity Health's Liquidation is Imminent," Lincoln Journal Star February 27, 2015.

7. Geoffrey A. Moore, *Crossing the Chasm, 3rd Edition: Marketing and Selling Disruptive Products to Mainstream Customers* (New York: Harper Collins Publishers, 2014).

8. Allan Toffler, *Future Shock*, (New York: Bantam Books, 1970)

9. Sydney J. Harris, *Quotable Quotes*, http://goodreads.com

10. Josh Linkner, "When to Pivot: 7 Signs Your Company is Dying," http://forbes.com, June 2013

11. Rick Warren, *The Purpose Driven Life: What on Earth Am I Here For?* (Grand Rapids: Zondervan, 2012).

12. Jeff Goins, *The Art of Work: A Proven Path to Discovering What You Were Meant to Do* (Nashville: Thomas Nelson, 2015).

13. Brennan Hussey, phone interview by author, April 30, 2015.

14. Zoher Kapasi, "Health Reform Law and its impact on Physical Therapists, Journal of the American Physical Therapy Association," Vol. 13, No.1, Fall 2010.

15. PwC Health Research Institute, "Healthcare's new entrants: Who will be the industry's Amazon.com?"

16. Thomas W. Malone, *The Future of Work* (Boston: Harvard Business School Publishing, 2004.

17. eMarketer Report, "Millennials in the Marketplace: A Generation Moving on Its Own Unpredictable Path." http://www.emarketer.com, June 6, 2013.

18. Sergio Pablos, *Despicable Me*, directed by Pierre Coffin (Santa Monica, CA Illumination Entertainment, 2007)

19. *Merriam-Webster Dictionary*, http://www.merriam-websterdictionary.com.

20. Paul Graham, "The High–Res Society," http://paulgraham.com, December 2008.

21. Ibid

22. Richard Afable M.D., "When I'm 64: How Boomers Will Change Healthcare," American Hospital Association, 2006.

23. Karen Litzy PT, phone interview by author, July 26, 2014.

24. Eric Ries, *The Lean Startup: How Today's Entrepreneurs Use Continuous Innovation to Create Radically Successful Businesses*, (New York: Crown Publishing, 2011).

25. Perry Marshall, *80/20 Sales and Marketing: The Defining Guide to Working Less and Making More*. (Entrepreneur Press, 2013).

26. J.R.R. Tolkien, *The Lord of the Rings*, directed by Peter Jackson (Los Angeles, CA New Line Cinema, 2001-2003).

# ABOUT THE AUTHOR

Paul Potter is a physical therapist and mentor who lives in Lincoln, Nebraska with his wife, who is also a therapist. They have four daughters. For more than 35 years he successfully managed his own private practice. He has authored the *Cash Therapy Practice: Professional Freedom in the New Healthcare Economy*. His website PaulPotterPT.com and his podcast "Functional Freedom" are dedicated to helping therapists build their dream practices.

Connect with Paul on his website or on Twitter @lifetouchpt. You can also get more free resources at PaulPotterPT.com/cash-therapy-practice.

PaulPotterPT.com

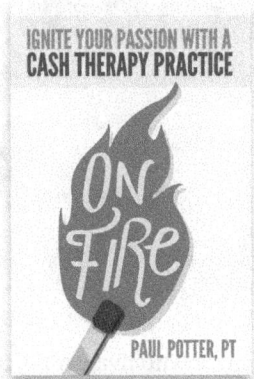

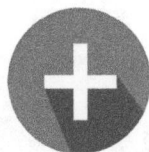

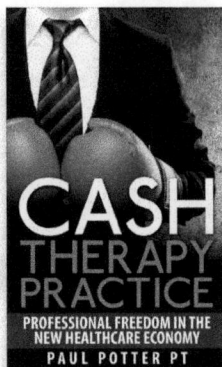

## DOWNLOAD YOUR FREE BOOK BONUSES

### GET STARTED TODAY

This book provides an honest discussion and practical advice to help you to succeed in the new healthcare economy. There is a lot of information to digest in these pages. To help you take action on this information, I've created several worksheets, checklists and resources. If you are serious about applying what you've learned in this book, download your free resources at www.PaulPotterPT.com/cashtherapypractice

I also recommend that you start right now. Building a successful practice is mostly learning by doing. The sooner you get started, the faster you'll grow your platform and your practice. I'm here to help. Please share your comments, ideas, questions and feedback by emailing heypaul@ paulpotterpt.com

### All You Have To Do is Go Here Now:

# PAULPOTTERPT.COM/CASHTHERAPYPRACTICE

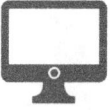

## Blog

I've started a blog and podcast to support therapists who want to create their dream practices. I'm building a community for therapists who want to take the best of the past and bring it into the opportunities of the new healthcare economy. Learn more at PaulPotterPT.com/cashtherapypractice.

## Updates

Sign up for free updates at PaulPotterPT.com and join the community.

## Share

If you've benefited from this book, please share it. You can link to it from you site, quote it and share it on your social media links. Please share your feedback with me at heypaul@PaulPotterPT.com

To Your Best Year Ever,
Paul Potter

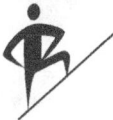

**PAUL POTTER PT**
START UP / STEP UP / **STAND OUT**

www.ingramcontent.com/pod-product-compliance
Lightning Source LLC
Chambersburg PA
CBHW061838220326
41599CB00027B/5331